Sameh Mezri

Sleep disorders in healthcare workers

Sameh Mezri

Sleep disorders in healthcare workers

ScienciaScripts

Imprint

Any brand names and product names mentioned in this book are subject to trademark, brand or patent protection and are trademarks or registered trademarks of their respective holders. The use of brand names, product names, common names, trade names, product descriptions etc. even without a particular marking in this work is in no way to be construed to mean that such names may be regarded as unrestricted in respect of trademark and brand protection legislation and could thus be used by anyone.

Cover image: www.ingimage.com

This book is a translation from the original published under ISBN 978-620-6-71527-6.

Publisher:
Sciencia Scripts
is a trademark of
Dodo Books Indian Ocean Ltd. and OmniScriptum S.R.L publishing group

120 High Road, East Finchley, London, N2 9ED, United Kingdom
Str. Armeneasca 28/1, office 1, Chisinau MD-2012, Republic of Moldova, Europe
Printed at: see last page
ISBN: 978-620-7-80227-2

TABLE OF CONTENTS

INTRODUCTION

Sleep is a vital need that takes up a third of a human being's existence. It is a period of rest lasting 6 to 8 hours per nycthemer, preferably taken during the night. It is essential to life, both physically and mentally. Sleep disorders are a real public health problem. They have a major impact on how individuals function, and on their social and professional lives, because of their considerable daytime consequences [1].Nearly a third of the population complains of a sleep disorder, and despite their high frequency, sleep disorders remain poorly identified. In fact, less than 20% of people with sleep disorders are correctly diagnosed and treated [2].However, certain work patterns deserve special attention because of the consequences they can have not only on the work itself but also on the worker. This is the case with shift work, which most often includes a night shift. Shift work has a direct and major impact on sleep. Between 60% and 70% of shift workers complain of sleep problems [3]. So while sleep influences productivity at work, in some cases it is the working conditions associated with shift work, particularly night work, that disrupt sleep quality. The impact of this can be significant, particularly for certain professions such as healthcare professionals whose work directly affects patient safety. Healthcare workers are among the most exposed to sleep disorders because they work atypical hours and against the biological clock. It is therefore necessary to study the impact of shift work, particularly night work by healthcare professionals, on sleep in order to develop a prevention strategy that limits the harmful consequences for health and the provision of care for patients. This is because, The epidemiology of sleep disorders is still poorly understood, and few studies, particularly in Tunisia, have looked at the evaluation of sleep problems in nursing staff as a function of their working habits. Hence our interest in carrying out this work.The aim of our study was to investigate the frequency of sleep disorders in healthcare workers performing shift work.

METHODS

1. Type of study and population studied

This is a descriptive cross-sectional study which took place in October 2023 at the main military training hospital in Tunis, targeting nursing staff working in shifts to ensure continuity of care.

1.1. Inclusion criteria

Our study included nursing staff (nurses/care assistants/anaesthetists/instrumentalists) who work in continuous shift mode with fixed successive shifts and who agreed to take part in the study.

1.2. Exclusion criteria

The following were excluded

✓ The doctors

✓ Administrative staff

✓ Care staff who work in shifts alternating between

✓ Professional activity < 3 months

2. Methods

2.1. Definitions

2.1.1. Shift and night work

Shift work is a form of work organisation in which teams work in succession to ensure the continuity of a service. The mode is said to be fixed when each team always occupies the same working time slot [4]. Under the French Labour Code, night work is defined as work performed between 9pm and 6am.

2.1.2. Sleep disorders

The International Classification of Sleep Disease established by the American Academy Of Sleep Medicine distinguishes several categories [5] :

- **Dyssomnias**: are characterised by abnormalities in the quantity or quality of sleep or sleep cycles. This disorder includes insomnia, hypersomnia, sleep disorders related to breathing and circadian rhythm disorders.

➢ Insomnia: This is a subjective feeling that covers difficulties in falling asleep: insomnia in falling asleep (considered when there is a latency of 45 minutes or more before falling asleep), insomnia in the middle of the night or during the night (considered when there are two or more night-time awakenings), waking up too early without being able to go back to sleep (early morning insomnia), or sleep that is not recuperative.

➢ Hypersomnias: An increase in sleep time. A distinction is made between pathological hypersomnias (primary or secondary) and induced hypersomnias.

➢ Sleep disorders related to breathing: these include central sleep apnoea syndromes (such as Cheynes-Stokes), obstructive sleep apnoea/hypopnoea syndromes and alveolar hypoventilation syndrome.

- **Parasomnias**: characterised by abnormal behavioural or physiological events occurring during sleep or during the sleep/wake transition.

-**Sleep disorders linked to abnormal movements: These are** relatively simple, stereotyped movements that occur during sleep.

-**Sleep disorders associated with pathologies.**

2.1.3. Excessive daytime sleepiness

The most common consequence of poor sleep. It is defined by real episodes of falling asleep, sometimes irresistible, more or less recuperative and unwanted. In our study, excessive daytime sleepiness (EDS) was assessed on the basis of the

Epworth scale included in the questionnaire, with a score greater than or equal to 10 [6].

✓ Score < 9 was considered as no sleep debt.

✓ Score between 10 and 14 is in favour of a sleep debt.

✓ A score of 15 or more indicates a highly probable sleep disorder.

2.1.4. Pichot fatigue scale

To assess fatigue in our participants, we used the Pichot scale. A total score of more than 22 was considered to indicate excessive fatigue [7].

2.1.5. Berlin Questionnaire

We used the Berlin questionnaire to screen for obstructive sleep apnoea syndrome (OSA). This questionnaire comprises three categories of questions and does not allow a diagnosis to be made, but does allow a risk to be classified and the need for polysomnography to be assessed. Two positive categories define a high risk of obstructive sleep apnoea syndrome [8].

2.1.6. Obesity

Obesity is defined by a Body Mass Index (BMI), calculated by dividing weight by height squared (kg/m^2), greater than or equal to 30 (kg/m^2). Overweight is defined as a BMI between 25 and 29.9 (kg/m^2).

2.2. Questionnaire

A questionnaire was distributed online to the hospital's healthcare staff. The questionnaire focused on the following themes (**appendix**):

✓ Characteristics of participants (age/ sex/ occupation/ habits (alcohol, tobacco, coffee, sleeping pills) / medical history.

✓ Characteristics of the workstation (Night or day worker /Seniority of work

/Work schedule /Seniority of work schedule/Personal choice of work schedule or imposed).

✓ Sleep studies (total sleep time/duration of sleep/naps/recovery sleep or not/sleep disorders (insomnia, hypersomnia, restless sleep).

✓ Assessment of daytime sleepiness using the Epworth scale.

✓ Assessment of fatigue using the Pichot score.

✓ Screening for sleep apnoea syndrome using the Berlin questionnaire.

2.3.Statistical analysis

The data were entered using Excel and analysed using SPSS. Our participants were divided into two groups according to whether they worked during the day or at night, in order to assess the impact of night shifts on sleep. For the descriptive study, we calculated simple frequencies and relative frequencies (percentages) for the qualitative variables. We calculated averages and determined extreme values for quantitative variables. For the analytical study, the Chi2 test was used to compare percentages of paired series, and the Student's t test was used to compare means. In all statistical tests, the significance level was set at 0.05.

3. References

For bibliographic research, the following databases were consulted: Elsevier Masson Consult (EMC), PubMed, Science direct; and the search engines Google® and Google Scholar®. Key words used: work, sleep disorder, healthcare staff, questionnaire, sleepiness, fatigue. Bibliographic references were managed using Zotero® software.

4. Ethical considerations

The purpose of the study was announced at the beginning of the questionnaire. Anonymity was maintained throughout the study and participants were not asked for any information about their identity.

RESULTS

1. Characteristics of the population studied

1.1. Socio-demographic data

The total number of participants included in our study was 60. The average age of our population was 38, with a minimum of 23 and a maximum of 57. The most common age group was between 20 and 30, accounting for 37% of participants. (Figure 1).There was a clear predominance of women: 38 women (63%) and 22 men (37%), with a sex ratio of 0.57.

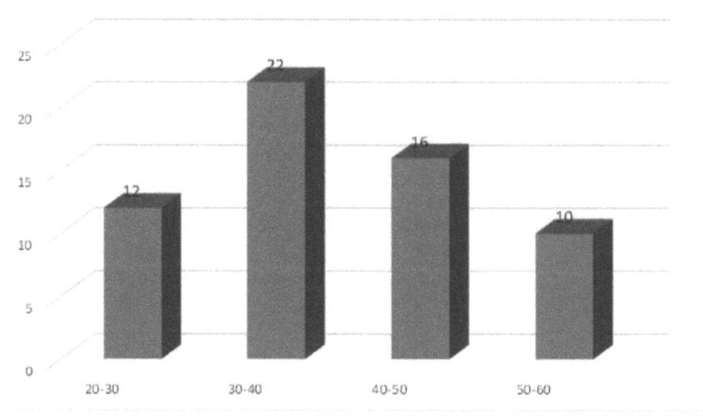

Figure 1: Breakdown of the study population by age group.

1.2. Breakdown by occupation

Sixty per cent (60%) of the participants were nurses (N=36) and the remainder (N=24) were healthcare assistants, anaesthesia technicians or instrument technicians. (Figure 2)

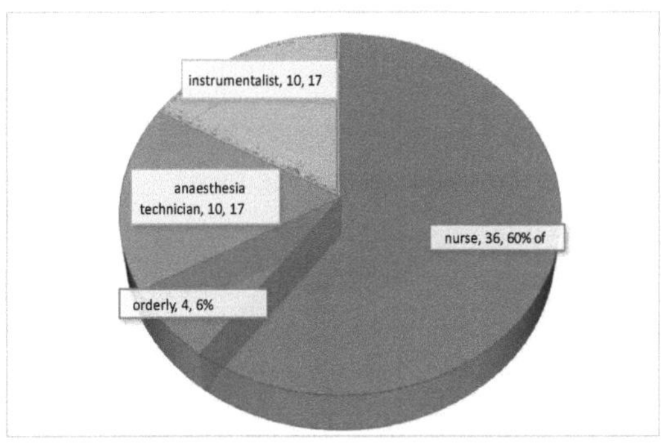

Figure 2: Breakdown of participants by profession

1.3. Lifestyle habits

Fifty participants were non-smokers and the prevalence of smoking was 17%. Only two of the nursing staff were alcoholics (3%).Ten per cent (10%) of participants reported using sleeping pills. All our participants were coffee drinkers, with an average of two cups of coffee a day and a minimum of one cup and a maximum of 4 cups a day.

1.4. Medical history

The participants' faults were investigated. Indeed, 20% of the nursing staff were hypertensive. However, there was no evidence of OSA. (Figure 3).

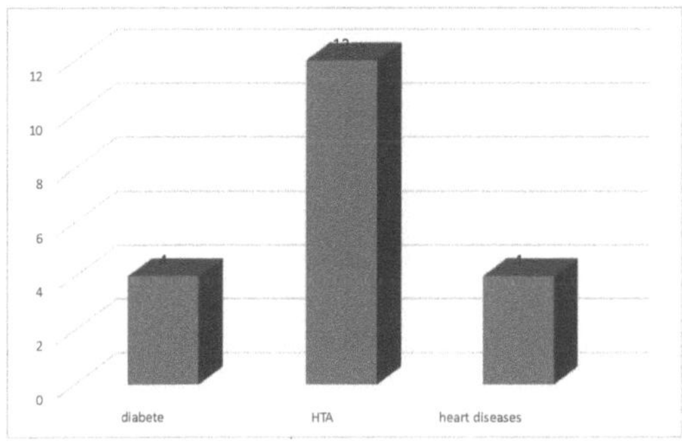

Figure 3: Participants' medical history

1.5. Body mass index

BMI ranged from 19 to 38 kg/m2, with an average of 25.5 ± 4.9 kg/m2. Obese patients represented 20% of our population. (Figure 4)

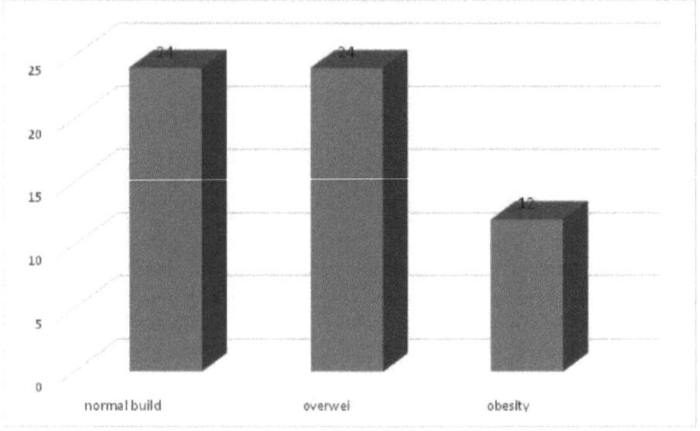

Figure 4: Breakdown by body mass index

2. Shift working conditions

2.1. Night or day worker status

The participants in our study were divided into two groups according to working hours: night workers (N=34) and day workers (N=26). (Figure 5)

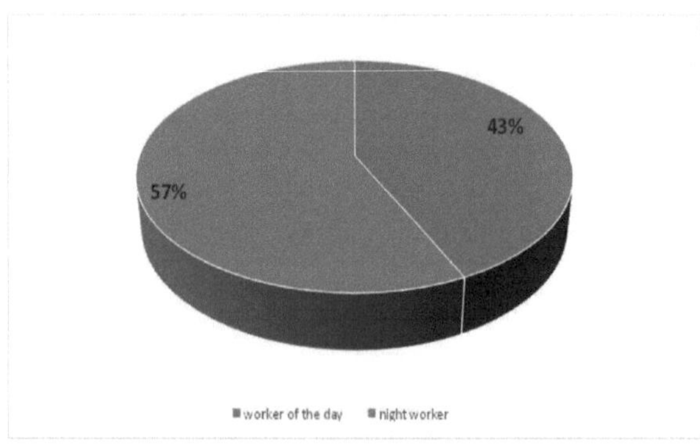

Figure 5: Breakdown of participants by working hours

Our participants were divided into night workers and day workers with the following characteristics: (Table I) We found that night shift workers were more obese (p=0.001).

Table I: Characteristics of workers by working hours

Day worker		Night workers	p
Average age	37.7 years old	38.8 years old	0,68
Consumption of sleeping pills	2 (8%)	4 (12%)	0,602
Coffee consumption per day	1,92	2,11	0,603
Obesity	O	12 (35%)	0,001

2.2. Working hours and seniority

Sixty-seven percent (67%) of the participants (N=40) chose the work schedule. For the others, the schedule was imposed by the needs of the department. In fact, 38% of day workers and 88% of night workers chose the work schedule, with a significant statistical relationship (p=0.000) (Figure 6).

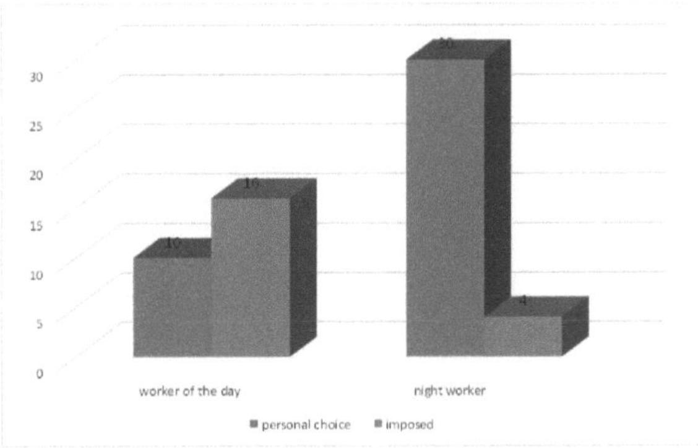

Figure 6: Breakdown of participants by choice of working hours

Sixty-seven percent (67%) of the nursing staff in our study had been working between one and 10 years (Figure 7).

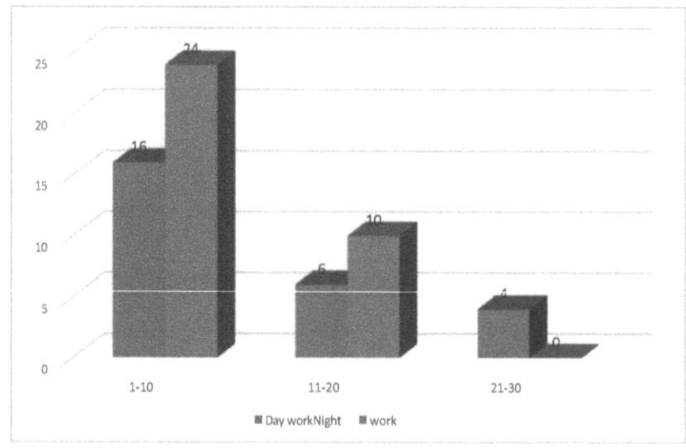

Figure 7: Breakdown of workers by length of service

3. Sleep studies

3.1. Quantitative study of sleep

3.1.1. Total sleep time

The average daily sleep time in our study was 6.7 hours, with a minimum of 5 hours and a maximum of 8 hours. The average sleep time for night workers was 6 hours per day, less than for day workers (7.5 hours per day), with a significant statistical relationship (p=0.000) (Figure 8).

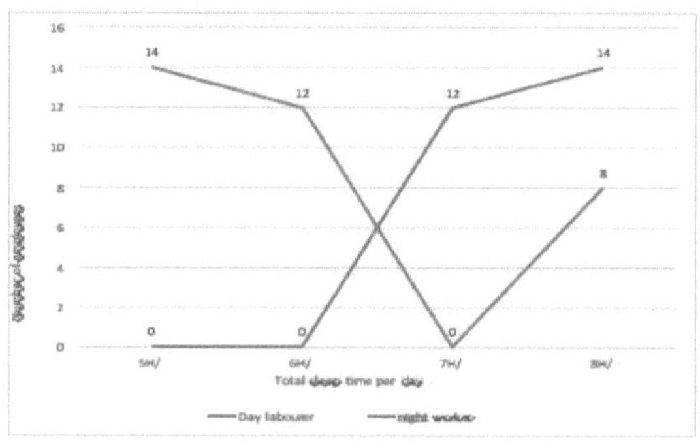

Figure 8: Quantitative study of sleep according to working hours

3.1.2. Time taken to fall asleep

In our study, the average time taken to fall asleep was 32 minutes, with a minimum of 5 and a maximum of 60 minutes.The average time taken to fall asleep for day workers was 26.3 minutes less than that for night workers, which was 36.8 minutes, with a significant statistical relationship (p=0.02). Night workers had more difficulty falling asleep. (Figure 9)

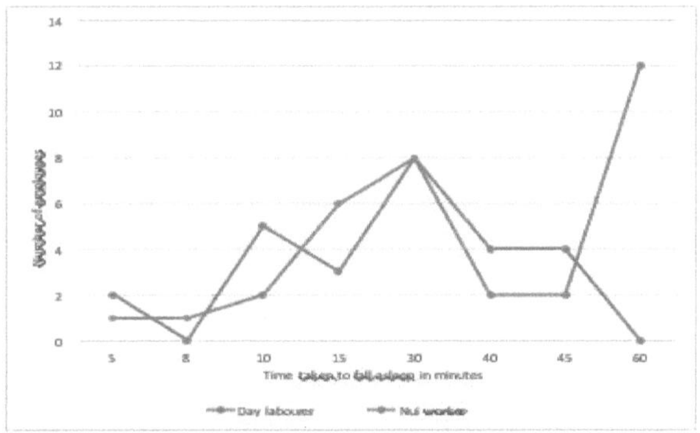

Figure 9: Study of sleepiness according to working hours

According to the average time spent asleep reported by our participants, 41% of night workers (N=14) and 15% of day workers (N=4) had insomnia on falling asleep.

3.2. Qualitative study of sleep

Sixty percent (60%) of the participants in the study declared that their sleep was not recuperative, including 71% of night workers (N=24) and 46% of day workers (N=12), with no significant statistical difference (p=0.056). Forty-three percent (43%) of the nursing staff in our study took a nap during the day, ten of whom were day workers (38%) and sixteen night workers (47%), with p=0.505 not significant.

3.3. Sleep disorders

According to the participants, 50% had sleep problems. In fact, 71% of night workers and 23% of day workers reported having sleep problems, with a significant statistical difference (p=0.001). The sleep disorders reported by night workers were insomnia (47%), hypersomnia (12%), or restless sleep (12%), while those reported by day workers were restless sleep (15%) and insomnia (8%). (Figure 10)

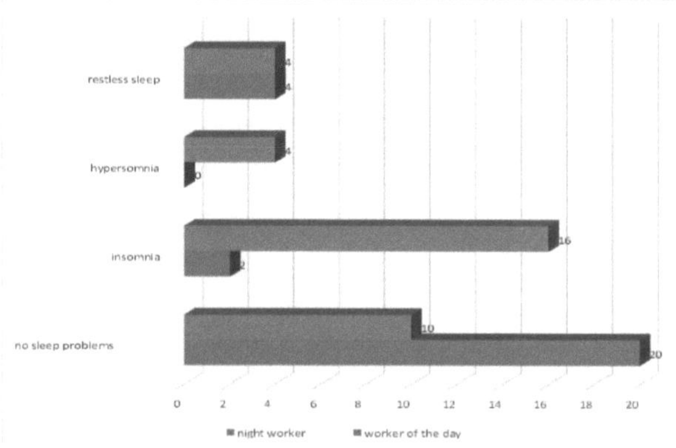

Figure 10: Breakdown of sleep problems experienced by healthcare workers

3.4. Sleep-disordered breathing

In our study, we used the Berlin questionnaire to screen for sleep apnoea syndrome. Twenty-five per cent (25%) of our participants (N=15) were at risk of sleep apnoea syndrome according to this Berlin score. Night workers were more at risk of OSA than day workers, with prevalences of 29% and 19% respectively, with no significant statistical relationship (p=0.367). (Table II)

Table II: Results of the Berlin questionnaire according to working hours

	Day labourer	Night workers
Category 1 positive	5 (19%)	14 (41%)
Category 2 positive	4 (15%)	11(32%)
Category 3 positive	5 (19%)	12(35%)
BERLIN SCORE	5 (19%)	10 (29%)

4. Impact of sleep on shift work

4.1. Epworth sleepiness scale

In order to measure any sleepiness during the day, we used the Epworth scale. The mean Epworth score in our study was 10.1, with a minimum of 7 and a maximum of 17.A study of daytime sleepiness based on this score showed that 38% of daytime workers and 77% of night-time workers had daytime sleepiness, with a significant statistical relationship (p=0.003). (Figure 11)

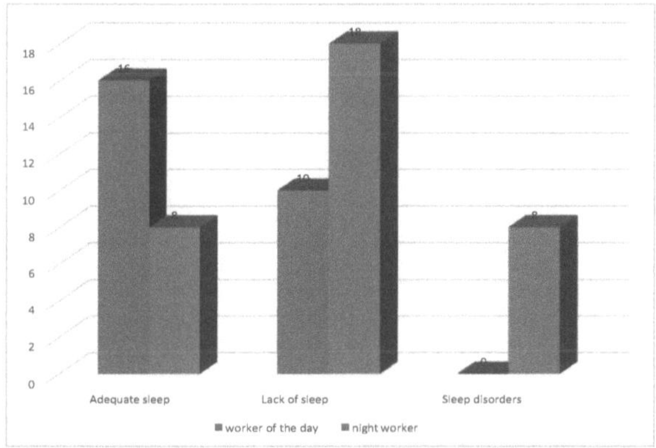

Figure 11: study of sleepiness using the epworth scale

4.2. Pichot fatigue scale

To assess fatigue in our study participants, we used the Pichot scale. The mean Pichot score in our study was 16.6, with a minimum of 7 and a maximum of 24. According to this score, no excessive fatigue was noted among daytime care workers, whereas 35% of night workers (N=12) had excessive fatigue, with a significant statistical relationship (p=0.001).

4.3. Concentration and memory problems

In our study, 45% of care workers reported concentration and memory problems, including 42% of day workers and 47% of night workers, with no significant statistical relationship (p=0.714). When the care staff taking part in the study were asked whether they had adopted sleep hygiene as part of their routine, 87% said no.

5. Summary

At the end of our work, our main results evaluating the impact of shift work by healthcare workers on sleep are set out in the following table: Table III.

Table III: Summary table of main results

	Day labourer	Night workers	p
Average sleep time	7.5 h/day	6h/day	p=0,000
Average time to sleep	26.3 minutes	36.8 minutes	p=0,02
Insomnia on falling asleep	4 (15%)	14(41%)	-
Insomnia	8%	47%	-
Hypersomnia	-	12%	-
Restless sleep	15%	12%	-
Sleep-disordered breathing (SDB)	19%	29%	p=0,367
Excessive daytime sleepiness	38%	77%	p=0,003
Excessive fatigue	0	35%	p=0,001
Concentration and memory problems	42%	47%	p=0,714

Our main results

Early diagnosis and appropriate management of sleep disorders in healthcare professionals is important and inevitably involves determining their frequency in relation to the work schedule. Hence our interest in carrying out this work, the main objective of which is to study the frequency of sleep disorders in healthcare workers performing shift work. This is a cross-sectional study carried out in October 2023 using an anonymous questionnaire distributed to health workers working in fixed shifts at the main military training hospital in Tunis.

We had 60 participants: 38 women (63%) and 22 men (37%). These participants were divided into two groups: 57% night workers (N=34) and 43% day workers (N=26). Sixty-seven percent (67%) of the participants (N=40) chose their work schedule. In fact, 38% of day workers and 88% of night workers chose the work schedule (p=0.000).The average sleep time for night workers was 6h/d, less than that for day workers (7.5h/d) with (p=0.000). However, the average time taken to fall asleep for day workers was 26.3 minutes less than that for night workers, which was 36.8 minutes, with a significant statistical relationship (p=0.02). Forty-one percent (41%) of night workers (N=14) and 15% of day workers (N=4) had insomnia on falling asleep. According to the participants, 50% (N=30) had sleep disorders. These problems were more pronounced among night workers than day workers, with a significant statistical difference (p=0.001).The sleep disorders reported by night workers were insomnia (47%), hypersomnia (12%), or restless sleep (12%), while those reported by day workers were restless sleep (15%) and insomnia (8%).A study of daytime sleepiness using the Epworth score showed that EDS was more prevalent among night staff than day staff, with a significant statistical relationship (p=0.003).According to the Pichot fatigue scale, excessive fatigue was noted only among night workers (35%), with a statistically significant difference (p=0.001). Twenty-five percent (25%) of our participants (N=15) were at risk of obstructive sleep apnoea syndrome according to the Berlin score. Night workers were more at risk of OSA than day workers, with prevalences of 29% and 19% respectively, with no significant statistical relationship (p=0.367). Concentration and memory problems were found in 42% of day workers and 47% of night workers, with no significant statistical difference (p=0.714).

Strengths and weaknesses of the study

Creating an online questionnaire is an advantage. It makes it easier to read, to access (via any digital medium), to complete and to collect data. However, the disadvantage of an online questionnaire is that a very large number of healthcare workers did not respond, either because they were not interested or because they did not receive the questionnaire. In fact, the size of the sample of participants was relatively small, making it impossible to provide meaningful responses on certain points. In addition, a sleep diary should have been added to the questionnaire, allowing a more precise analysis of sleep-wake rhythm disorders and a better analysis of the impact of sleep disorders on daytime vigilance.

DISCUSSION

1. Sleep and wellness

Sleep is a period of rest lasting 6 to 8 hours per nycthemer, preferably taken during the night and allowing physical and psychological recovery and structuring of the knowledge acquired during wakefulness. Sleep is therefore an essential physiological phase.

The ideal length of a night's sleep is one that allows you to feel "The result is a 'refreshed' night's sleep, so that you're fit and efficient the next morning. The majority of the French population needs between 7 and 8 hours of sleep (Baromètre Santé 2020, 12th edition) [1].

During this phase, the body takes the opportunity to restore, renew and repair the tissues and functions required during wakefulness. Lack of sleep has an impact on the quality of work and, conversely, the conditions in which waking activities are carried out (physical activity, tension, stress, etc.) affect sleep quality [5].

Quality sleep means falling asleep quickly, sleeping deeply and waking up rarely and briefly during the night. Sleep quality can be affected by factors such as stress, anxiety, sleep disorders and sleep habits [1]. The average daily sleep time in our study was 6.7 hours, with a minimum of 5 hours and a maximum of 8 hours.

2. Shift work and sleep

Shift work has a direct and major impact on sleep. Between 60 and 70% of night workers complain of sleep problems. Their sleep is insufficient, unsatisfactory and poorly restorative. Night work therefore leads to a reduction in the quality and quantity of sleep [1,4,9,10].Night work requires the individual to work during a period of deactivation and to sleep during the activation phase. Lack of exposure to daylight throws internal clocks out of sync and disrupts biological rhythms. Night work can have a more or less serious impact on employees' health, ranging from sleep disorders to the risk of cancer [11,12].

2.1.Quantitative sleep disorders

Irregular working hours or prolonged periods of work disrupt our circadian rhythm and make it difficult to fall asleep or stay asleep [9,10].

Several studies have shown that night work leads to sleep and alertness disorders. In fact, the sleep of night-shift workers was shorter than normal, and this duration was reduced by 1 to 1.5 hours [4,13,14,15]. This was shown in our study, where the average sleep time for night shift workers was 6 hours per day, less than for day shift workers (7.5 hours per day), with a significant statistical relationship (p= 0.000).

Any type of shift work can lead to sleep loss, but this is particularly pronounced in atypical schedules, including night shifts, since night workers go to bed when their diurnal rhythm favours wakefulness [14,16].

Working at night means going against the rhythm of other people's lives: when you get home from work, you try to enjoy your family and friends instead of sleeping to recuperate. Even if it's only for a few minutes, sleep time is shortened and can turn into sleep debt, with numerous repercussions on health: stress, irritability, concentration problems [10,17].

2.2.Sleep quality disorders

Shift work is perceived as altering the quantity and quality of sleep. Employers say that they sleep less and less well, wake up more often during the night and get less sleep. at night, waking up more difficult [4]. In our study, 60% of participants reported having non-restorative sleep, including 71% of night workers and 46% of day workers (p=0.056).

Several studies have used the Pittsbugh Sleep Quality Index (PSQI) to assess sleep quality. This questionnaire covers seven areas: subjective sleep quality, sleep onset latency, usual sleep duration, usual sleep efficiency, sleep disorders, use of sleeping pills, and daytime dysfunction over the last month. Among these studies, Dai C et al [18] in China included 865 nurses divided into 2 groups: the 1st group worked at night and the 2nd group worked in the morning. The authors found that poor sleep quality was more frequent in night staff than in day staff (84.2% vs 68.4%, p<0.001) [18]. Unfortunately, we did not use this score in our study.In a Tunisian study carried out at the Mongi Slim Hospital, 158 paramedical staff were interviewed (46.2% were nurses, 23.4% were manual workers, 19% were senior technicians and 11.4% were orderlies, midwives and physiotherapists). Sleep disorders were detected in 40.5

OSA in 24% of cases [19]. In our study, 50% of healthcare workers had sleep disorders, including 71% of night workers and 23% of day workers, with a significant statistical difference (p=0.001).Insomnia is a subjective experience that includes difficulty falling asleep, frequent waking up at night or waking up too early without being able to go back to sleep, or sleep that is not recuperative [5]. In the general population, the prevalence of insomnia varies from study to study and from country to country. Studies conducted in Japan, the United States and Western Europe show insomnia rates ranging from 10% to 48%. Insomnia was the most common sleep disorder (44%) in a Tunisian study [20]. Using the Bergen Insomnia Scale, a Norwegian study involving 2059 nurses showed that nurses who worked nights suffered more insomnia than nurses who had never worked nights [14]. Indeed, some studies report positive associations between former night work and chronic insomnia [21]. In a study of sleep disorders associated with shift work, Haile KK et al [22] found a prevalence of insomnia of 25.6% among 422 nurses working at the Federal Hospital in Adis Ababa (Ethiopia). In another study conducted in Brazil involving intensive care unit nursing staff, a prevalence of insomnia of 42% was described [23]. In our study, insomnia was the most reported sleep disorder among 47% of night workers and

8% of day workers.The type of insomnia in nursing staff is rarely specified in studies [20].

The use of sleeping pills is certainly an important indicator of the severity of insomnia. Our study showed that sleeping pills were taken in 10% of cases. This result is close to that described by El Machrou H [24] (5.7%) and Elbiaze M [25] (6%). In a Tunisian study including 118 hospital staff working at the Farhat Hached University Hospital and the Sahloul University Hospital in Sousse, a higher proportion of night staff than day staff had difficulty falling asleep (46.3% versus 22.2%, p<0.01), with poorer sleep quality compared to their day colleagues [26].

A Moroccan study of 69 nurses working at night showed that 54% had difficulty falling asleep [15]. In our study, the average time taken to fall asleep for day workers was 26.3 minutes less than that for night workers, which was 36.8 minutes (p=0.024). In fact, 41% of of night workers (N=14) and 15% of day workers (N=4) had insomnia on falling asleep. Research has shown that night workers often have difficulty falling asleep during the day, leading to sleep deprivation and chronic fatigue. Over time, they can develop shift-work disorder, a condition characterised by insomnia when trying to sleep and excessive fatigue when at work [4].

2.3.Risk of sleep apnoea syndrome

Some studies have looked at the prevalence of obstructive sleep apnoea syndrome in healthcare professionals, showing that this category of staff is more exposed to the risk of OSA than the general population [13].

Snoring is the most reported sign of OSA. In a Greek study including 444 nurses working in 2nd and 3rd line hospitals, the prevalence of snoring was 29.8% [27].

A French study of 773 participants working in a university hospital who volunteered to answer the Berlin questionnaire found that the prevalence of subjects at high risk of OSA was 22.4% among nursing staff and 21.4% (17-

26%) among shift workers [13].

A study of healthcare professionals in Morocco showed a 50% prevalence of OSAS in subjects classified as being at high risk of OSAS by the Berlin questionnaire [28].

In Germany, a study of nurses working shift work showed a prevalence of OSA of 43% using the Berlin questionnaire and polysomnography [29].

Paciorek et al show that the apnoea-hypopnoea index during polysomnography was higher in shift workers than in controls [30].

Excessive smoking and changes in eating habits during night work encourage the development of obesity, which is the main risk factor for the onset of OSA. A Tunisian study showed that metabolic syndrome was diagnosed in 51.2% of shift workers and 27.2% of non-shift workers, with a significant difference (p<10-3) [31].

The potential link between disturbances in sleep-wake rhythm and the development of obesity appears complex, as obesity itself may be an aggravating factor in sleep disorders. It seems that obesity may produce an alteration in deep slow-wave sleep. What's more, the stress generated by night shifts in hospitals and the workload carried out by a small number of nursing staff have a direct impact on sleep quality on the one hand, and on food consumption on the other, leading to the development of obesity. A vicious circle is forming [4].

By forcing workers to sleep and work at times when their bodies are not always ready to do so, night shift work also leads to cardiovascular disorders, depressive and neurotic nervous disorders often associated with over-consumption of alcohol and tranquillisers, which further disrupt sleep [19].

In the light of these studies, it is therefore interesting, on the one hand, to propose screening for OSA among employees of a healthcare establishment and, on the other hand, to use the Berlin questionnaire as a screening tool.

2.4. Excessive daytime sleepiness

Care staff are affected by temporary or repeated night shifts. Sleep disorders can also result in excessive daytime sleepiness. This sleepiness may be secondary to sleep deprivation, fragmented sleep or genuine sleep disease [32].

We opted for the Epworth scale, which is admittedly a subjective questionnaire, but it would be reliable for diagnosing all chronic sleepiness. It also has the advantage of being quick, easy to complete and inexpensive. A review of the literature shows that the prevalence of EDS in nursing staff differs from one study to another, depending on the cutoff point of the Epworth scale used to define this symptom. In a questionnaire survey of 1102 nurses in China [33], the prevalence of EDS diagnosed in the case of an Epworth score $\geq$ 14 was 16.1%. The determinants of EDS in this study were depression, anxiety, insomnia and shift work [33]. However, the prevalence of EDS in a Tunisian study was 41.6% in nursing staff, based on the Epworth score ($\geq$10) [20].

In addition, work-related stress, which increases during shift work in hospitals, can also cause EDS. In our study, daytime sleepiness was more common among night nurses than day nurses (77% versus 38%, with a significant statistical relationship p=0.003).EDS was significantly more common in staff whose work required sustained attention (90.6% vs. 9.4% with p=0.03). This factor was implicated in 2 Moroccan studies [24,25].

The consumption of stimulants does not seem to have an impact on the frequency of EDS according to a Tunisian study [20], while El Machrouh H [24] found that coffee consumption is a protective factor against EDS.

In a multivariate study, the authors showed that short sleep duration was a risk factor for EDS [34]. On the other hand, experience of shift work was negatively associated with sleep problems in a Norwegian study [35].

2.5. Chronic fatigue and unrefreshing sleep

Nursing staff seem to choose night work for a variety of reasons: more free time during the day, greater autonomy and responsibility in their work, a better working atmosphere, and a higher income [36]. However, nurses who work fixed night shifts say that they have to do more physical work because they have to provide care that is generally given to nursing assistants during the day. Lower staffing levels at night, isolation, lack of communication with daytime teams and a lack of recognition for their work all contribute to the perceived hardship of night work or feelings of isolation in the workplace [37].

Sleep disorders and chronic fatigue are frequently reported by night shift workers. Night workers (especially women) sleep for shorter periods and their sleep is of poorer quality. Family commitments and conditions that are not conducive to sleep during the day reduce the quality and quantity of sleep for night workers, who accumulate a chronic lack of sleep over time. The increase in accidents at work and traffic accidents on the way home from work are consequences of this lack of sleep [17,37].

Sleep disorders resulting from poor sleep quality can have serious consequences for both the individual and the hospital, in terms of absenteeism, lack of concentration, memory problems, irritability, stress, reduced decision-making capacity, lateness and problems with work colleagues [4].

3. Prevention and recommendations

Night work is undeniably physically and mentally demanding. It is therefore important to take measures to minimise the negative impact of night work on the sleep of care staff, such as the introduction of a sleep routine and practising stress management techniques. It's also important to limit yourself to a reasonable pace of work and to set regular hours that aren't too intense [12].

3.1. Sleep hygiene

Sleep habits are a key element in good sleep, which is why we recommend :

•**Get at least 7 hours' sleep during the day: getting** a good night's sleep when it's light outside can be a challenge. To get enough sleep each day, it's advisable to take naps whenever you feel the need.

•**Adapting exposure to light:** the biological clock is regulated by exposure to light. When you return from night work, you need to limit your exposure to light as much as possible by making sure you filter out external sources of light (double curtains, sleep mask, limiting exposure to screens to at least 1 hour before bedtime, etc.). Conversely, before going to work, you should try light therapy, particularly in winter when it gets dark earlier, to balance your biological clock as much as possible.

•**Test melatonin-based dietary supplements** certain dietary supplements based on melatonin, lemon balm extract, California poppy and pale rose powder are beneficial for encouraging relaxation after a night's work.

•**Creating an optimal sleep environment:** noise can also disrupt sleep and increase the time it takes to fall asleep. Poor soundproofing, the family environment, notifications and phone calls can all have a major impact on sleep quality. Earplugs can also be used to block out outside noise.

•**A healthy lifestyle means** limiting stimulating activities, avoiding caffeine, alcohol and nicotine before bedtime, and avoiding hypnotic drugs to help you sleep.

•**In the event of drowsiness,** it is essential to recognise the signs of drowsiness at the wheel or at work and not hesitate to stop and sleep for 15-20 minutes. In the event of excessive daytime sleepiness and in the absence of sleep deprivation, a sleep disorder should be investigated by consulting a specialist.

3.2.Prevention

Shift and night work must be covered by the Labour Code. Management must be advised and supported by a number of preventive measures [12,36].

•Preventive measures relating to work organisation

-Setting up regular schedules and organising time for exchanges between teams

-Arrange the time system so that it interferes as little as possible with workers' lives.

-Prioritise workers who are willing and able to ensure business continuity.

-Provide break times by adapting the work premises.

•Preventive measures for workers

-Night workers are subject to appropriate individual monitoring by an occupational health professional during an information and prevention visit at intervals not exceeding 3 months.

-Employees are advised to eat a balanced diet, take part in sporting activities, get a good night's sleep and get used to taking micro-naps.

CONCLUSIONS

Sleep is a period of rest lasting 6 to 8 hours per nycthemer, preferably taken during the night, and allowing physical and psychological recovery and structuring of the knowledge acquired during wakefulness. However, certain working conditions can disrupt this physiological process.During shift or night work, the biological clock is disrupted. This disruption has an impact on sleep and alertness, increasing the risk of accidents, and can also lead to inattention in the workplace, increasing the number of professional errors. Healthcare workers are the most exposed to this type of work.The aim of this study was to investigate the frequency of sleep disorders in healthcare workers performing shift work.We had 60 participants: 38 women (63%) and 22 men (37%). These participants were divided into two groups: 57% night workers (N=34) and 43% day workers (N=26). Sixty-seven percent (67%) of the participants (N=40) chose the work schedule.The average sleep time for night workers was 6 hours per day, less than for day workers (7.5 hours per day), with a significant statistical relationship (p=0.000). However, the average time taken to fall asleep for daytime workers was 26.3 minutes less than that for night-time workers, which was 36.8 minutes, with a significant statistical relationship (p=0.02). In fact, 41% of night workers (N=14) and 15% of day workers (N=4) had insomnia on falling asleep.Sixty percent (60%) of the participants in the study said that their sleep was not recuperative. According to the participants, 50% (N=30) had sleep disorders. In fact, 71% of night workers and 23% of day workers reported having sleep disorders, with a significant statistical difference (p=0.001). The sleep disorders reported by night workers were insomnia (47%), hypersomnia (12%), or restless sleep (12%), while those reported by day workers were restless sleep (15%) and insomnia (8%).Twenty-five percent (25%) of our participants (N=15) were at risk of sleep apnoea syndrome according to the Berlin score. Night workers were more at risk of OSA than day workers, with prevalences of 29% and 19% respectively, with no significant statistical relationship (p=0.367).The study of daytime sleepiness based on the Epworth score showed that 38% of daytime workers and 77% of night-time workers suffered from daytime sleepiness, with a significant statistical relationship (p=0.003).According to the Pichot fatigue scale, no excessive fatigue was noted among daytime care staff, whereas 35% of night workers (N=12) were excessively fatigued, with a significant statistical relationship (p=0.001). In conclusion, working life and sleep are closely linked. Based on the results of this study, it is important to maintain good quality sleep in order to perform well at work. To minimise the impact of hospital night shifts on sleep, you need to adopt healthy sleep habits such as: regular working hours, a bedtime ritual, no physical activity for two hours before bedtime, invest in quality bedding and sound/light insulation in the bedroom. Obviously, you should avoid all screens in bed, and avoid taking stimulants at least 5 hours before bedtime, which will improve sleep quality and minimise the harmful effects on health. In addition, it is essential to improve night-time working conditions in hospitals by insisting on the importance of rest conditions, not forgetting regular medical monitoring of workers on night shifts by occupational medicine and screening for sleep disorders and EDS in the elderly. care staff, with particular attention paid to the risk of accidents in the workplace.

REFERENCES

1. Chennaoui M, Léger D. Sleep and the consequences of sleep deprivation: definitions and generalities. Def Natl. May 2022;(1):13-21.

2. Ohayon MM. Prevalence and comorbidity of sleep disorders in general population. Rev Prat. 2007 Sep;57(14):1521-8.

3. Rohmer O, Bonnefond A, Muzet A, Tassi P. Study of the sleep/wake rhythm, general motor activity and eating behaviour of obese shift workers: the example of nurses. Trav Hum. May 2004;67(4):359- 76.

4. Vallery G, Hervet C. Impact de diverses modalités organisationnelles du travail shift sur le sommeil, les comportements alimentaires, la vie sociale et familiale : le cas du personnel soignant en milieu hospitalier français. Interdisciplinary Perspectives on Work and Health. [On-line]. Feb 2005 [Accessed 28 Oct 2023]. Available at URL: https://journals.openedition. org/pistes/1055?lang=en

5. Sateia MJ. International classification of sleep disorders-third edition: highlights and modifications. Chest. 2014 Nov;146(5):1387-94.

6. Johns MW. A new method for measuring daytime sleepiness: the epworth sleepiness scale. Sleep. 1991 Dec;14(6):540-5.

7. Centre Du Sommeil. Pichot fatigue scale [Online]. Dec 2019 [Accessed 28 Oct 2023]; [1 page]. Available from URL: https://centre- sommeil-respire.fr/wp-content/uploads/2019/12/Echelle-de-fatigue-de- Pichot.pdf

8. Minh HT, Bich HN X. Role of Berlin questionnaire in screening of obstructive sleep apnea syndrome. J Fran Viet Pneu. 2012 Oct;3(9):26-31.

9. Hicklin D, Schwander J. Shift work and sleep. Praxis. 2019 Jan;108(2):119-24.

10. Boucetta N, Alaoui ME, Laafou M, Rouahi N. The impact of shift work on the health and well-being of health professionals at the health care centre. hospitalier provincial de Tétouan en 2021. Revue des Sciences Infirmières et Techniques de Santé. Feb 2022;1(1):36-43.

11. Cousin S. Night work: a high price to pay for health. [Online]. June 2019 [Accessed 28 Oct 2023]. Available from URL: http://www.remede. org/documents/night-work-a-high-price-to-pay-for-health.html

12. s. n. Theses on night work. 1989 [cited 31 Oct 2023]; Available from: https://www.e-periodica.ch/digbib/view?pid=rss-001:1989:81::273

13. Cadelis G, Fayad Y Monteagudo OE. Prevalence of symptoms and risk of obstructive sleep apnea syndrome assessed by the Berlin questionnaire among professionals of a health facility. Rev Epidemiol Sante Publique. 2016 Dec;64(6):405-14.

14. Øyane NF, Pallesen S, Moen BE, Akerstedt T, Bjorvatn B. Associations between night work and anxiety, depression, insomnia, sleepiness and fatigue in a sample of Norwegian nurses. PLoS One. Jul 2013;8(8):e70228.

15. Lghabi M, Allouche W, Benali B, El Kholti A. Impact of night work on the health of nurses. Arch Mal Prof. May 2018;79(3):419.

16. Montplaisir J, Infante Rivard C. Troubles du sommeil et de la vigilance chez les travailleurs hospitaliers ayant une expérience passée : horaires alternants jour/soir/nuit [On line]. June 1988 [Accessed 28 Oct 2023]. Available from URL: https://www.irsst.qc.ca/recherche-sst/projets/projet/i/303/n/troubles- du-sommeil-et-de-la-vigilance- chez-les-travailleurs-hospitaliers- ayant-une-ence-passee-horaires-alternants-jour-soir-nuit-0084-0010

17. Cheyrouze M, Barthe B. Night work in 12 hours: a "work scenario" developed by nurses in an intensive care unit. Activities. [Online]. Apr 2018 [Accessed 28 Oct 2023];15(1). Available at URL: https://journals.openedition.org/activites/3073?lang=en

18. Dai C, Qiu H, Huang Q, Hu P, Hong X, Tu J, et al. The effect of night shift on sleep quality and depressive symptoms among chinese nurses. Neuropsychiatr Dis Treat. 2019 Feb;15:435-40.

19. Brahim D, Snene H, Rafrafi R, Salah NB, Blibech H, Mehiri N, et al. Sleep disorders and psycho-affective problems in paramedical personnel working an atypical schedule. Rev Mal Respir. 2021 Feb;38(2):147-56.

20. Fahem N. Prevalence of sleep disorders in nursing staff [dissertation: medicine]. Tunis: University of Tunis El Manar; 2019.

21. Ingre M, Akerstedt T. Effect of accumulated night work during the working lifetime, on subjective health and sleep in monozygotic twins. J Sleep Res. 2004 Mar;13(1):45-8.

22. Haile KK, Asnakew S, Waja T, Kerbih HB. Shift work sleep disorders and associated factors among nurses at federal government hospitals in Ethiopia: a cross-sectional study. BMJ Open. 2019 Aug;9(8):e029802.

23. Guerra PC, Oliveira NF, Terreri MT, Len CA. Sleep, quality of life and mood of nursing professionals of pediatric intensive care units. Rev Esc Enferm USP. 2016 Apr;50(2):279-85.

24. El Machrouh H. The prevalence of sleep disorders among nursing staff at the CHR of Tetouan. Sidi Mohamed Ben Abdellah University, Faculty of Medicine and Pharmacy; 2017.

25. Elbiaze M, El Otmani FZ, Benjelloun M, Labyad S, Serraj M, Bouchra A, et al. The prevalence of excessive daytime sleepiness and its relationship with shift work among nursing staff at the Hassan II University Hospital in Fez. Sleep Medicine. Mar 2017;14(1):45.

26. Debbabi F, Chatti S, Magroun I, Maalel O, Mahjoub H, Mrizak N. Night work: its repercussions on the health of hospital staff. Arch Mal Prof. Oct 2004;65(6):489-92.

27. Alexandropoulou A, Vavougios GD, Hatzoglou C, Gourgoulianis KI, Zarogiannis SG. Risk assessment for self reported obstructive sleep apnea and Excessive daytime sleepiness in a Greek nursing staff population. Medicina. 2019 Aug;55(8):468.

28. Laraqui O, Laraqui S, Manar N, Caubet A, Verger C, Laraqui CH. Screening and symptoms of obstructive sleep apnea-hypopnea syndrome in a population of healthcare professionals in Morocco. Arch Mal Prof. Apr 2013;74(2):178-85.

29. Geiger Brown J, Rogers VE, Han K, Trinkoff A, Bausell RB, Scharf SM. Occupational screening for sleep disorders in 12-h shift nurses using the Berlin

questionnaire. Sleep Breath. 2013 Mar;17(1):381-8.

30. Paciorek M, Korczyński P, Bielicki P, Byśkiniewicz K, Zieliński J, Chazan R. Obstructive sleep apnea in shift workers. Sleep Med. 2011 Mar;12(3):274- 7.

31. Kacem I, Maoua M, Hasni Y, Kalboussi H, Hafsia M, Souguir S, et al. Evaluation of the risk of metabolic syndrome among shift workers in Tunisia. East Mediterr Health J. 2019 Nov;25(10):677-85.

32. Hausser Hauw C. Sleep disorders: excessive daytime sleepiness and insomnia. EMC - AKOS (Traité de médecine) 2008;3(1):1-9 [Article 1-0730].

33. Chen L, Luo C, Liu S, Chen W, Liu Y, Li Y, et al. Excessive daytime sleepiness in general hospital nurses: prevalence, correlates, and its association with adverse events. Sleep Breath. 2019 Mar;23(1):209-16.

34. Chaiard J, Deeluea J, Suksatit B, Songkham W, Inta N. Short sleep duration among Thai nurses: influences on fatigue, daytime sleepiness, and occupational errors. J Occup Health. 2018 Sep;60(5):348-55.

35. Bjorvatn B, Dale S, Hogstad Erikstein R, Fiske E, Pallesen S, Waage S. Self-reported sleep and health among Norwegian hospital nurses in intensive care units. Nurs Crit Care. 2012 Jul;17(4):180-8.

36. Chaouch N, Mechergui N, Aissi W, Essid D, Khemila T, Ladhari N. Effects of alternate shift work on quality of life and alertness in Tunisia. Sante Publique. Nov 2020;31(5):623-31.

37. Neves D. Night work and nurses' health [dissertation: psychology]. Lausanne: University of Lausanne; 2014.

APPENDIX

Sleep memory questionnaire Impact of shift work on sleep

I/Characteristics of the population

-Age

-Gender

-Profession

-HabitsAlcohol yes/no tobacco yes/no Consumption of coffee no. of cups per day Consumption of sleeping pills yes/no

-Medical history High blood pressure (balanced or not) Diabetes Dyslipidemia

Cardiovascular disease Obesity (BMI weight/height squared) OSA if yes (how long ago, type of treatment)

II shift work

-Night/day worker

-Length of service

-Working hours

-Length of service

-Personal choice of working hours yes/no

II/Sleep study

-Total sleep time per day in hours

-Time taken to fall asleep in minutes

- Do you take a nap (yes or no) if yes duration in minutes

- do you sleep well? yes or no

-Do you have sleep problems? insomnia/hypersomnia/disability to fall asleep/restless sleep

-Epworth Sleepiness Scale

To help you assess whether you might feel drowsy during the day, here are some relatively common situations in which we ask you to assess the risk of nodding off. If you haven't recently been in one of these situations, try to imagine how it might affect you.

To answer, use the following scale, circling the most appropriate number for each situation: 0 = no chance of dozing off or falling asleep

1 = low chance of falling asleep

2 = average chance of falling asleep

3 = high chance of falling asleep Chance of falling asleep :
1/Chassis reading 0 1 2 3

2/Watching television 0 1 2 3

3/Sitting, inactive in a public place (cinema, theatre, meeting) 0 1 2 3
4/Passenger in a car (or public transport) driving non-stop for an hour 0 1 2 3

5/Extended in the afternoon when circumstances permit 0 1 2 3

6/Sitting talking to someone 0 1 2 3

7/Calm down after an alcohol-free lunch 0 1 2 3

8/In a car that has been stationary for a few minutes 0 1 2 3

TOTAL Score=

-Pichot Fatigue Scale

Among the following eight propositions, determine which best correspond to your condition by assigning a score between 0 and 4: (0 = Not at all; 1= A little; 2 = Moderately; 3= Very much; 4 = Extremely)

1/I lack energy. 0 1 2 3 4

2/Everything takes effort 0 1 2 3 4

3/I feel weak in certain parts of my body................0 1 2 3 4

4-I have heavy arms or legs 0 1 2 3 4

5/I feel tired for no reason 0 1 2 3 4

6I want to lie down and rest.................................. 0 1 2 3 4

7-I find it hard to concentrate.................................0 1 2 3 4

8/I feel tired, heavy and stiff.................................. 0 1 2 3 4

Your Score : A total > 22 is in favour of excessive fatigue

-Risk of OSA (Berlin score)

The Berlin questionnaire is used to screen for sleep apnoea syndrome. This questionnaire cannot be used to make a diagnosis, but it can be used to classify risk and assess the need for polysomnography.

Category 1: Snoring

1) Do you snore? yes / no / don't know

If you don't snore, go on to question 5.

2) Is your snoring?

Slightly louder than your breathing. As loud as your voice when you speak. Louder than your voice when you speak.
Very noisy, you can be heard in neighbouring rooms.

3) How often do you snore? Almost every night.
3 to 4 nights per week.

1 to 2 nights per week.

1 or 2 nights per month.

4) Has your snoring ever bothered anyone else? yes/no

5) Have you ever noticed that you stop breathing while you sleep?

Almost every night. 3 to 4 nights a week.

1 to 2 nights per week.

1 or 2 nights per month.

Never or almost never at night.

Category 2: Drowsiness

6) How often do you feel tired or worn out after a night's sleep?

Almost every morning. 3 to 4 mornings a week.

1 or 2 mornings a week. Never or almost never.

7) Do you feel tired, weary or unwell when you're awake?

Almost every day. 3 to 4 days a week.

1 or 2 days a week.

1 or 2 days a month. Never or almost never.

8) Have you ever dozed off or fallen asleep at the wheel of your vehicle? yes/no

9) If so, how often does this happen to you? Almost every day.

3 to 4 days a week.

1 or 2 days a week.

1 or 2 days a month. Never or almost never.

Category 3: Risk factors

10) Do you suffer from high blood pressure? yes / no / don't know

11) I.M.C. $\geq$ 30 ? yes / no

Interpretation :

Categories 1 and 2 are positive from a score of 2 (answer in red), Category 3 from a score of 1.

Two positive categories define a high SAS risk.

-Do you have problems with memory and concentration at work? yes / no

-Have you adapted your sleep hygiene? yes/no

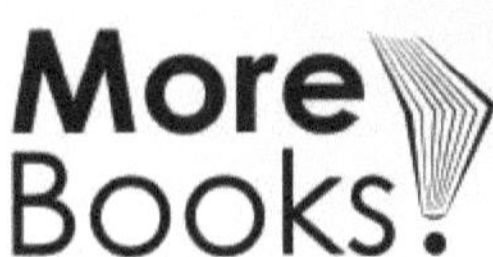

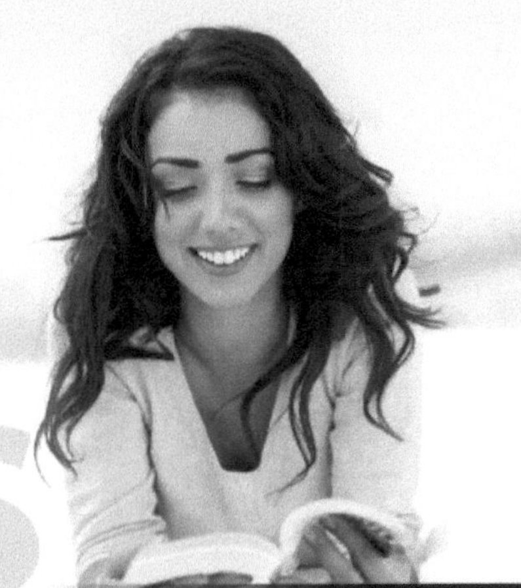

Buy your books fast and straightforward online - at one of world's fastest growing online book stores! Environmentally sound due to Print-on-Demand technologies.

Buy your books online at
www.morebooks.shop

Kaufen Sie Ihre Bücher schnell und unkompliziert online – auf einer der am schnellsten wachsenden Buchhandelsplattformen weltweit! Dank Print-On-Demand umwelt- und ressourcenschonend produziert.

Bücher schneller online kaufen
www.morebooks.shop

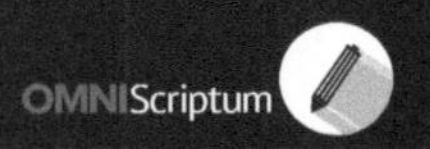

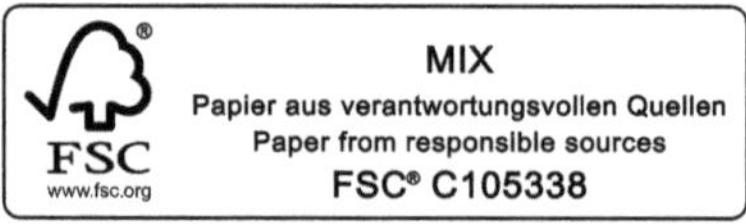

Printed by Books on Demand GmbH, Norderstedt / Germany